# This book Belongs To:

-------------------------------------------------------------

-------------------------------------------------------------

**Affirmations** are positive statements that are repeated to oneself in order to encourage a specific mindset or belief. They are typically used to promote self-confidence, motivation, and a positive outlook on life. Affirmations are often used in self-help and personal development practices to reprogram negative thought patterns and replace them with more positive ones. The idea is that by repeating affirmations regularly, an individual can change their subconscious beliefs and attitudes, which can in turn have a positive impact on their thoughts, feelings, and actions.

# I am grateful for all I have

# I provide excellent care to my patients.

# I listen to my patient's concerns and give them my full attention.

"

I show kindness and compassion to every patient.

"

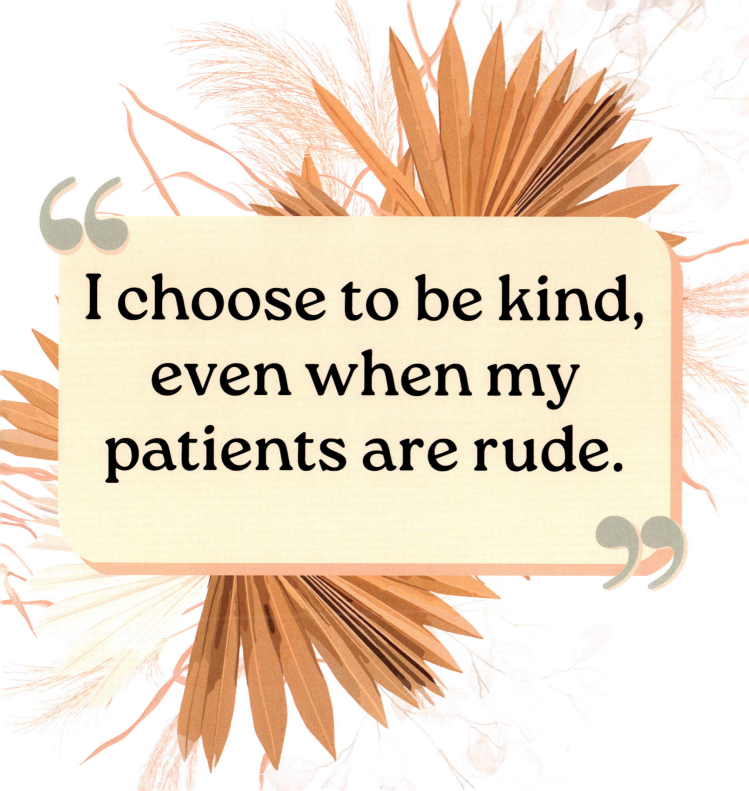

"I choose to be kind, even when my patients are rude.

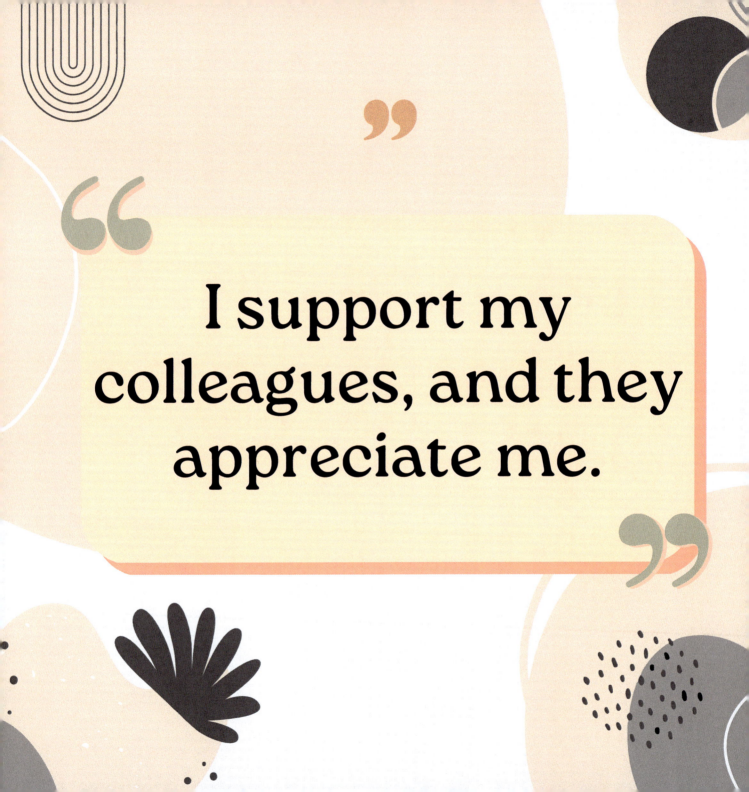

I support my colleagues, and they appreciate me.

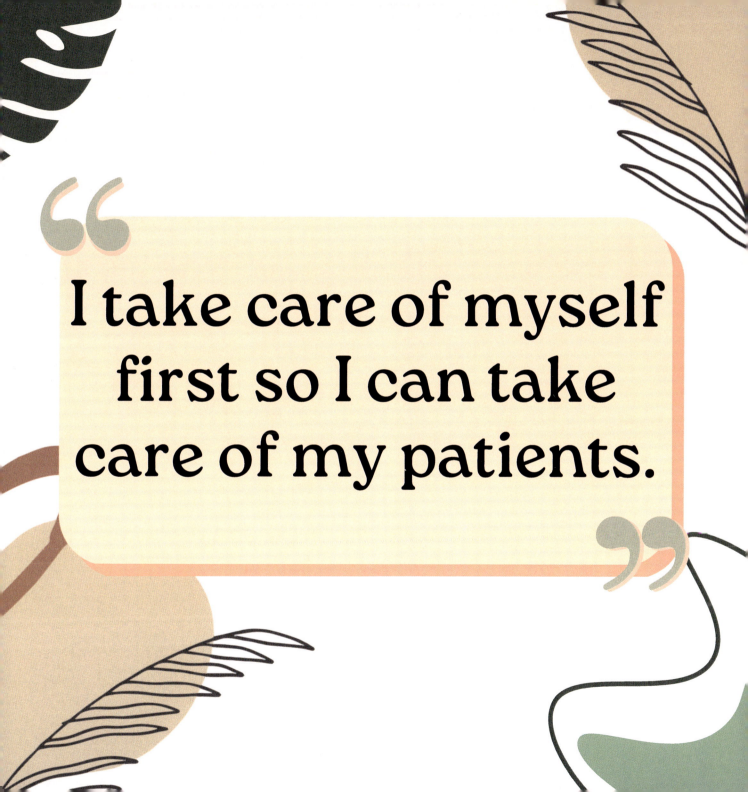

I take care of myself first so I can take care of my patients.

# I rest when I can so I can perform at my best.

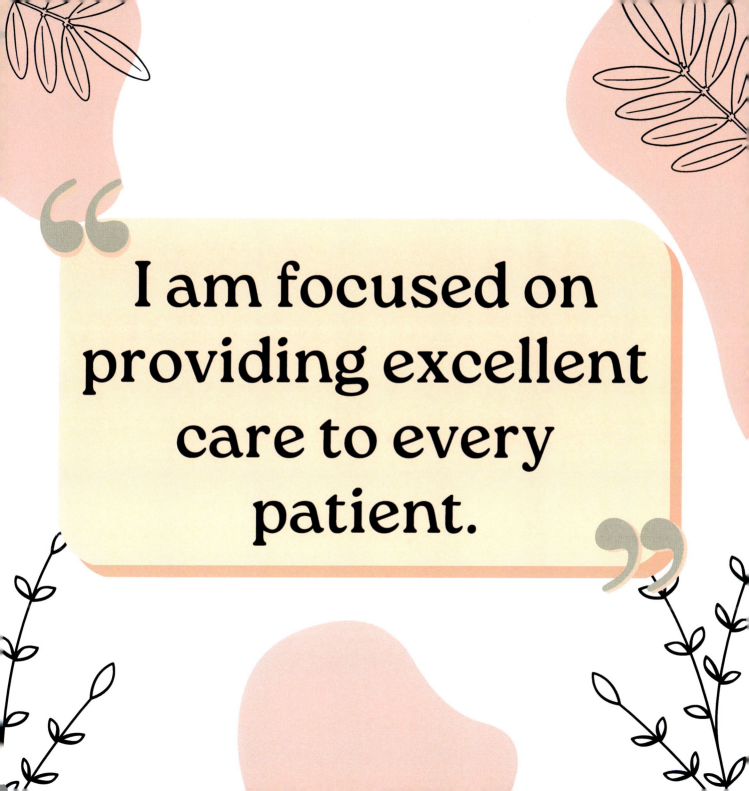

I am focused on providing excellent care to every patient.

"I always look for opportunities to learn. There is always something new to learn."

"
I am an important
and valued member
of my patient's
medical team.
"

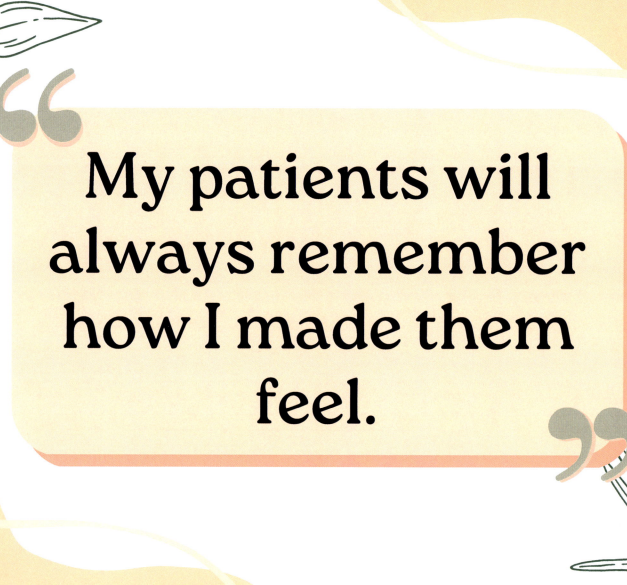

My patients will always remember how I made them feel.

# My patients trust me to care for them.

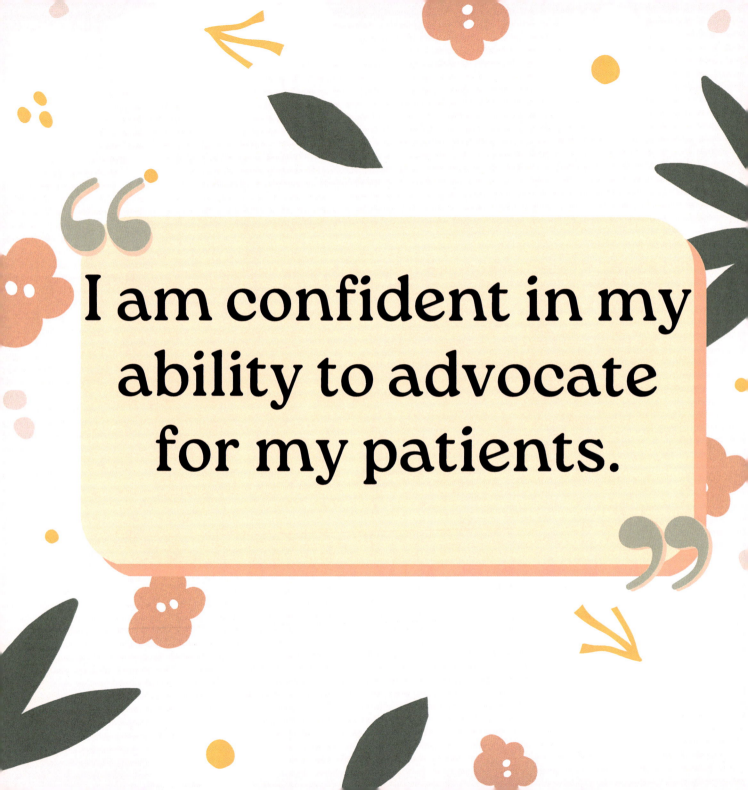

"I am confident in my ability to advocate for my patients."

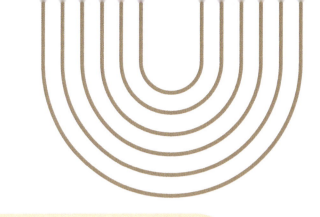

# I focus on the things that are within my control.

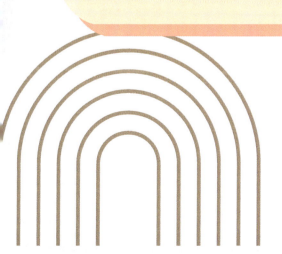

"

Every day is different, I love the challenges each day presents.

"

# I make a difference in the lives of my patients.

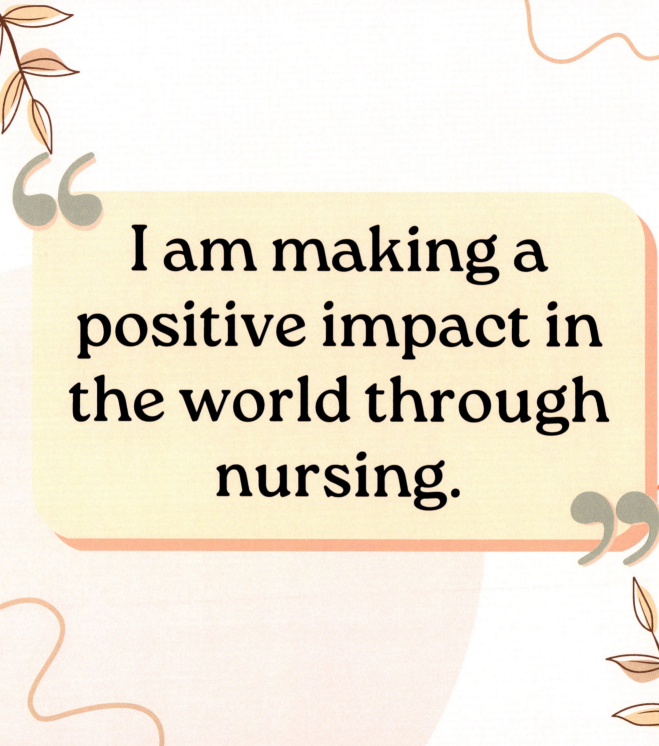

I am making a positive impact in the world through nursing.

"

I seek out mentors who I trust and who are passionate teachers.

"

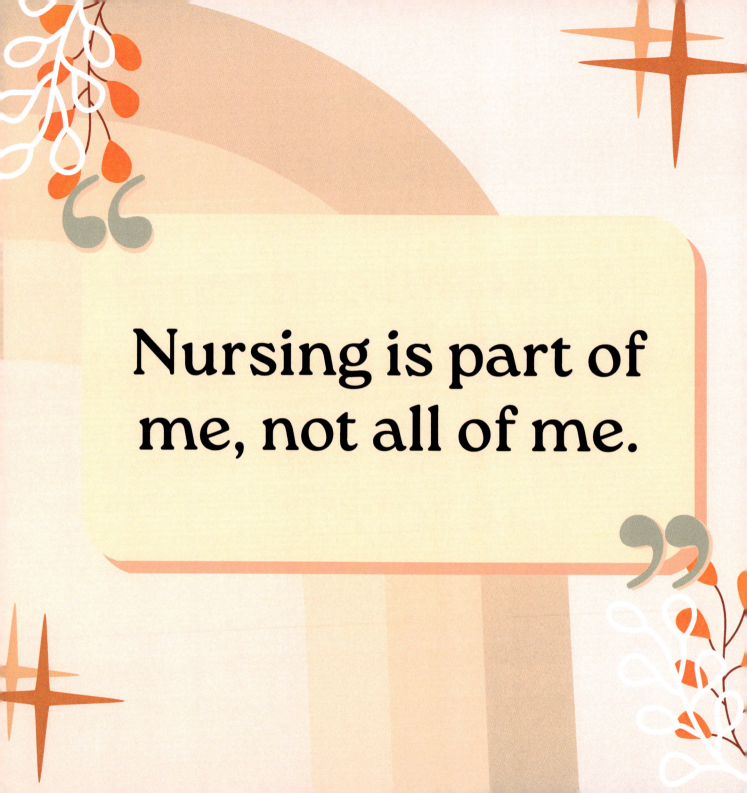

"

I set healthy boundaries between my work and home life.

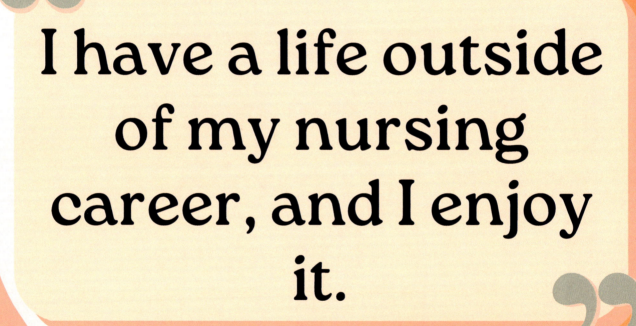

"I have a life outside of my nursing career, and I enjoy it.

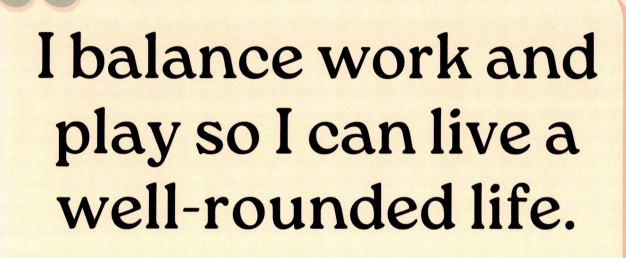

"I balance work and play so I can live a well-rounded life."

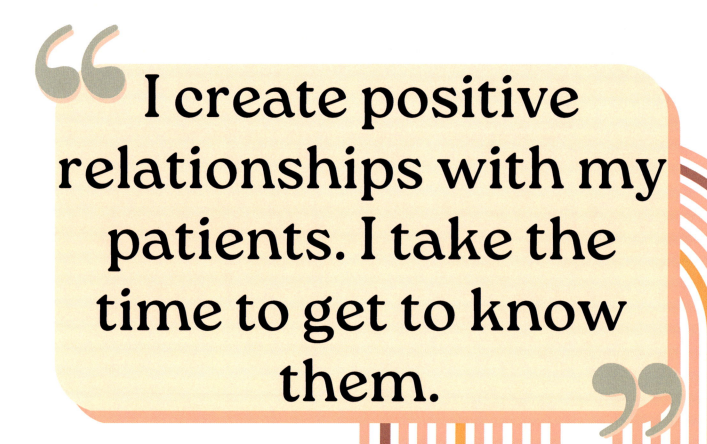

"I create positive relationships with my patients. I take the time to get to know them."

# I treat my patients the way I would want to be treated.

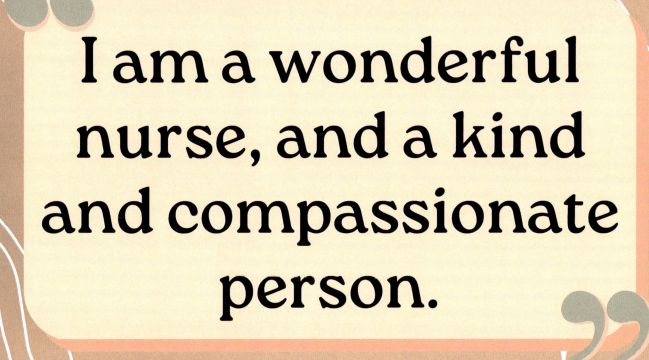

I am a wonderful nurse, and a kind and compassionate person.

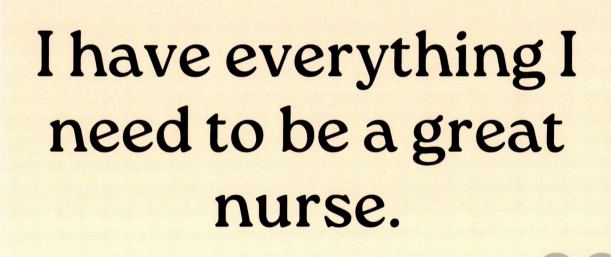

I have everything I need to be a great nurse.

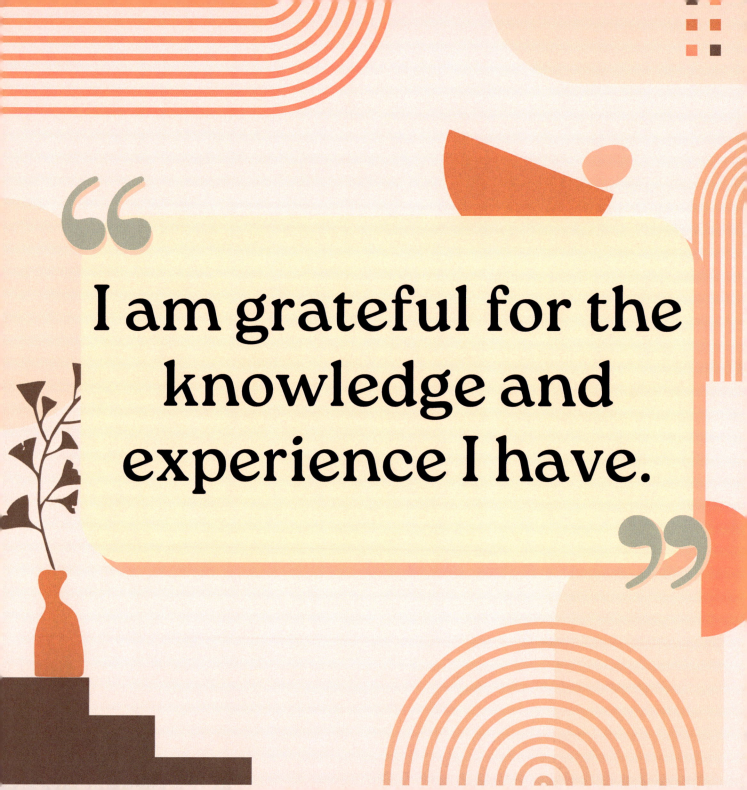

I am grateful for the knowledge and experience I have.

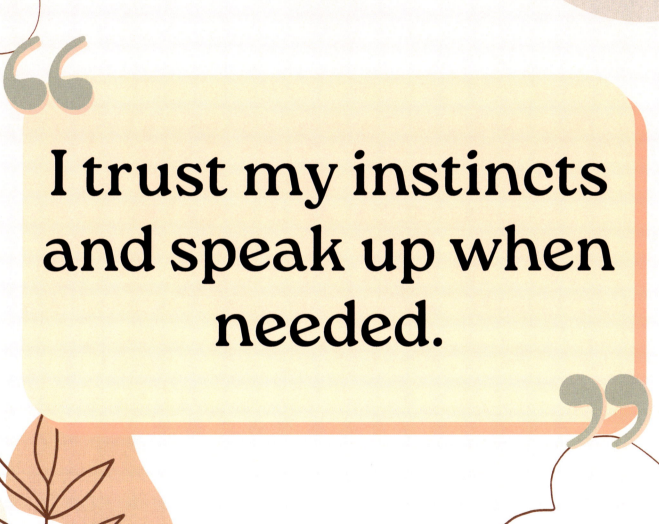

I trust my instincts and speak up when needed.

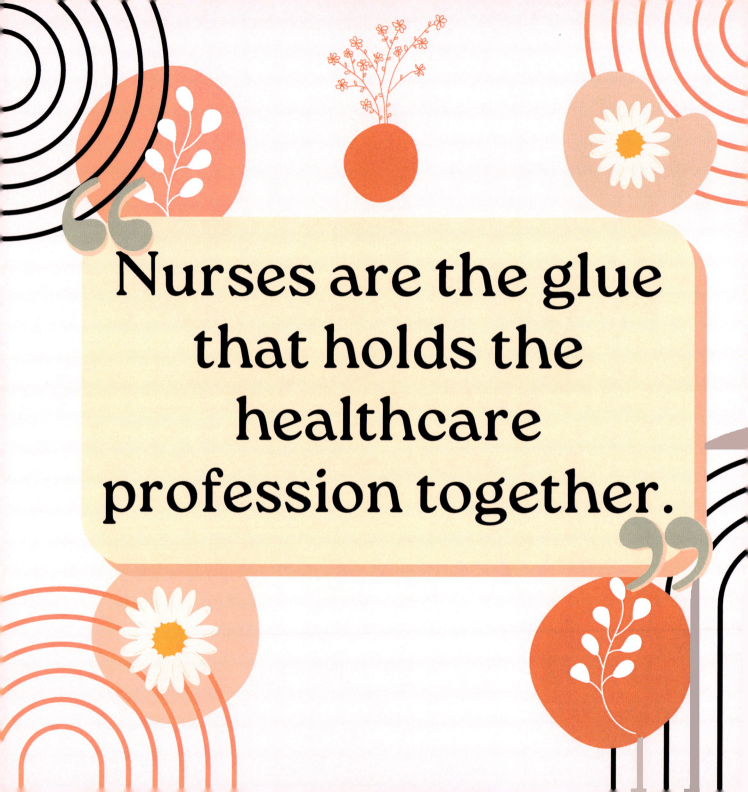

"Nurses are the glue that holds the healthcare profession together."

"My patients are my top priority. I always put their needs first.

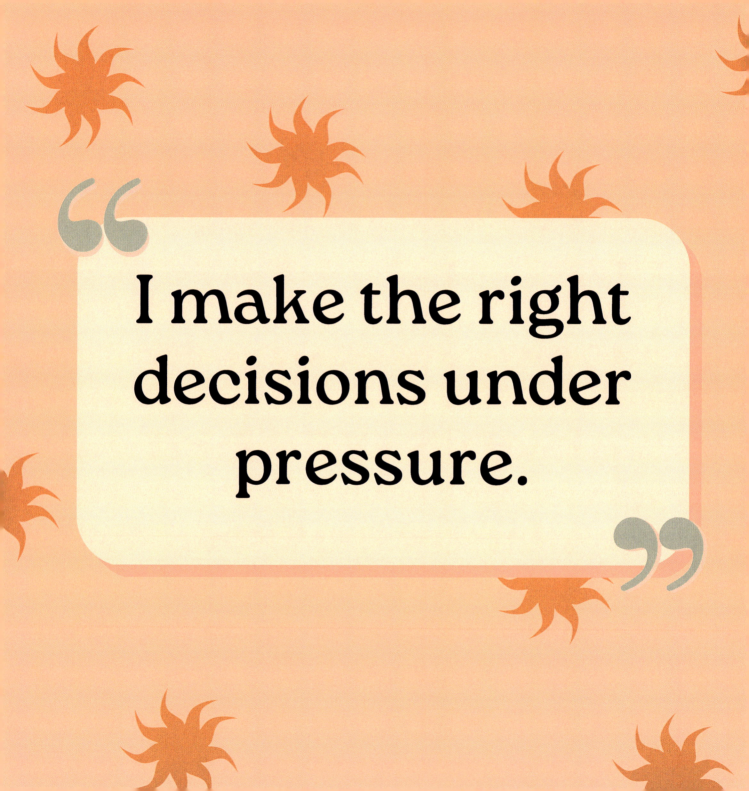

I make the right decisions under pressure.

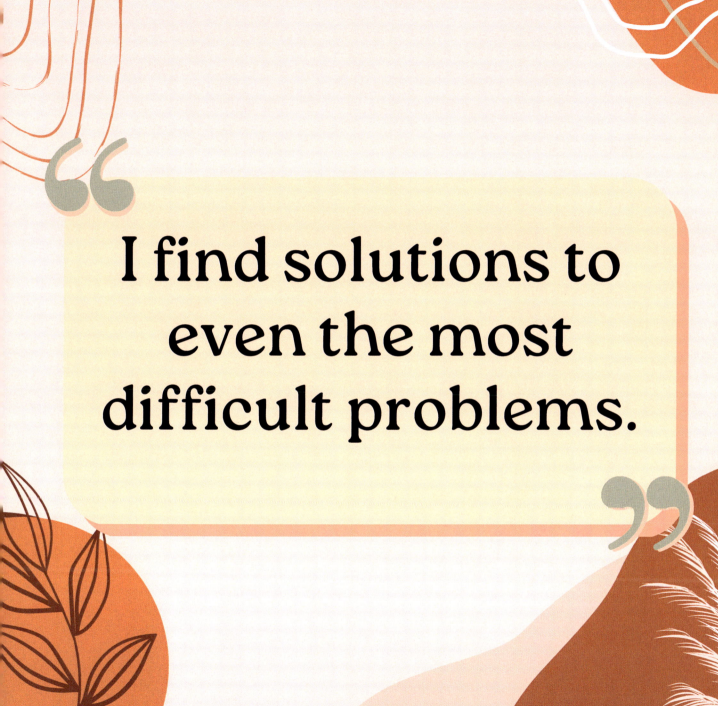

I find solutions to even the most difficult problems.

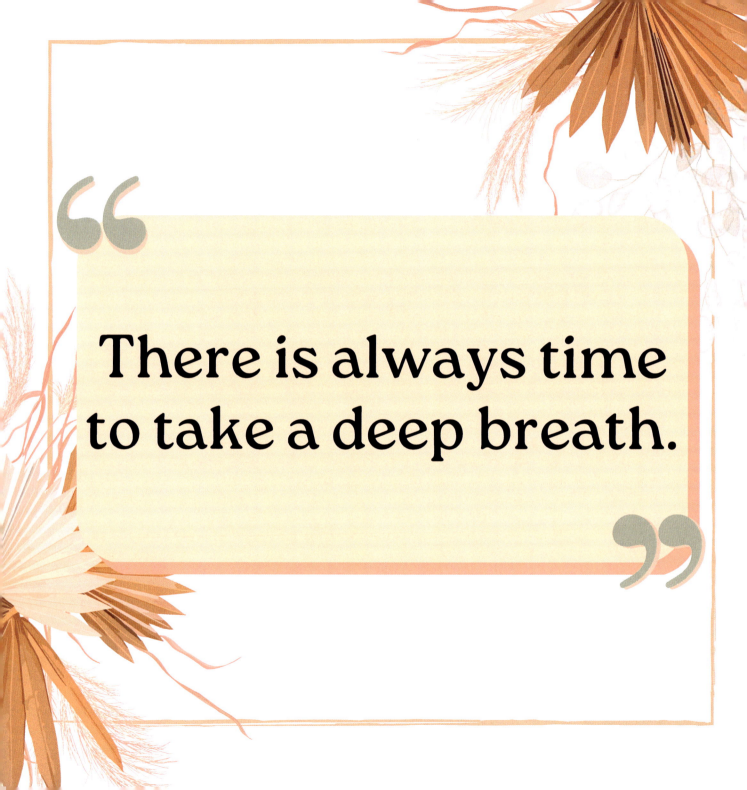

There is always time to take a deep breath.

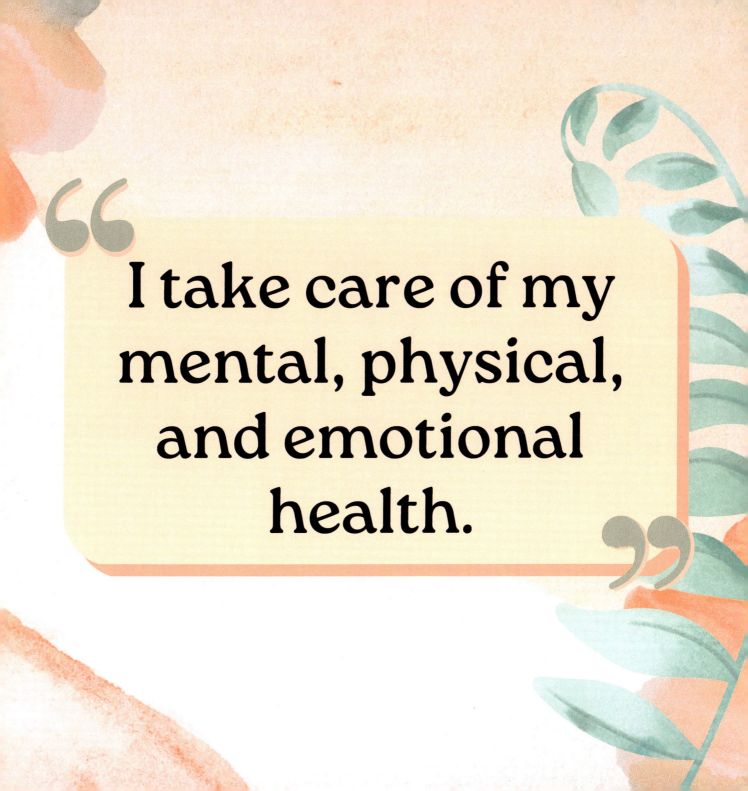

I take care of my mental, physical, and emotional health.

"It is okay for me to take a break and remove myself from stressful situations.

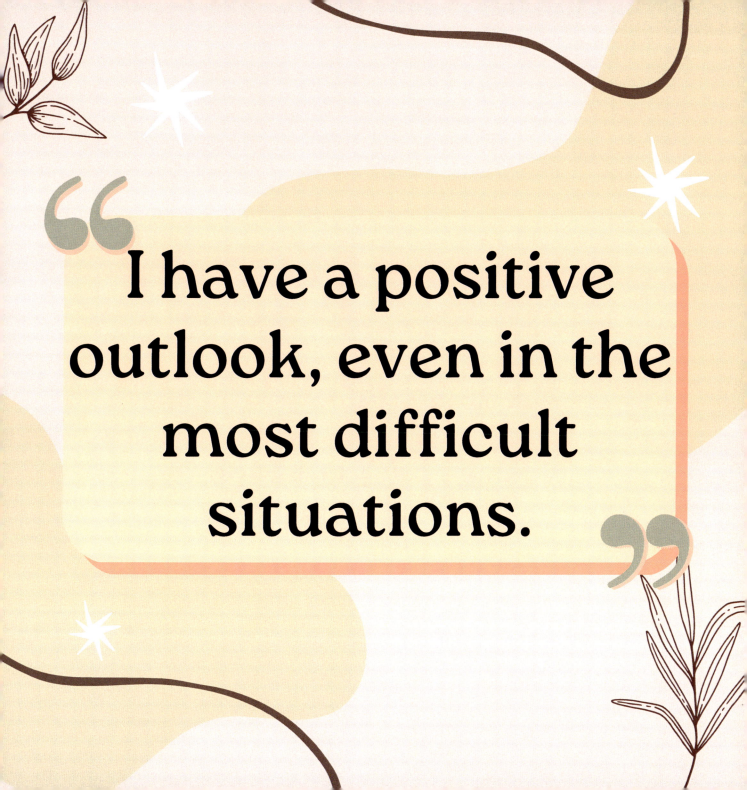

I have a positive outlook, even in the most difficult situations.

"

I choose to see the good in people and situations.

"

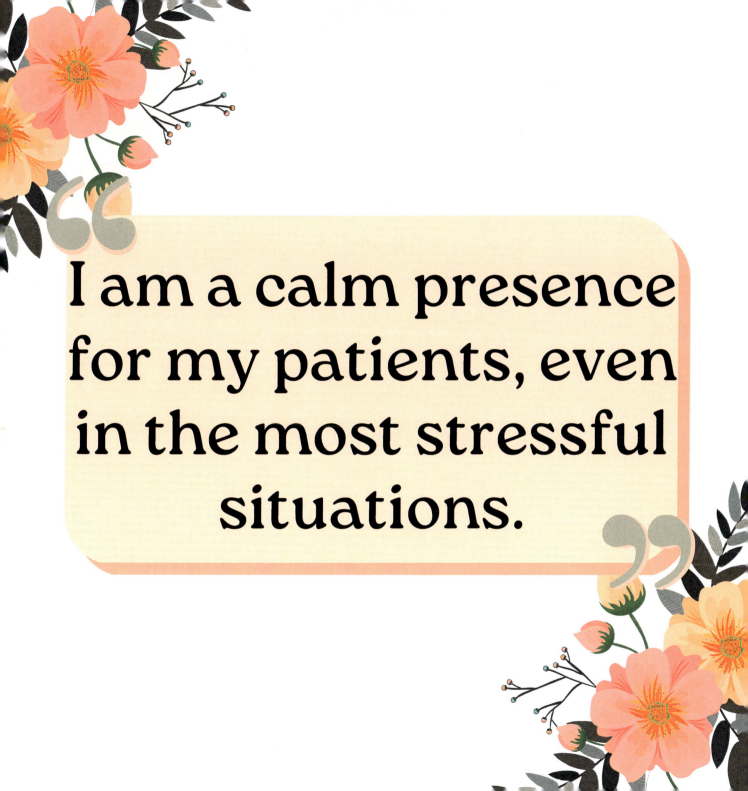

I am a calm presence for my patients, even in the most stressful situations.

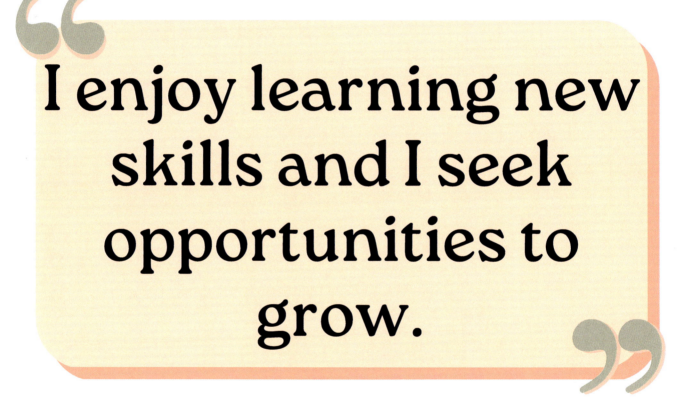

I enjoy learning new skills and I seek opportunities to grow.

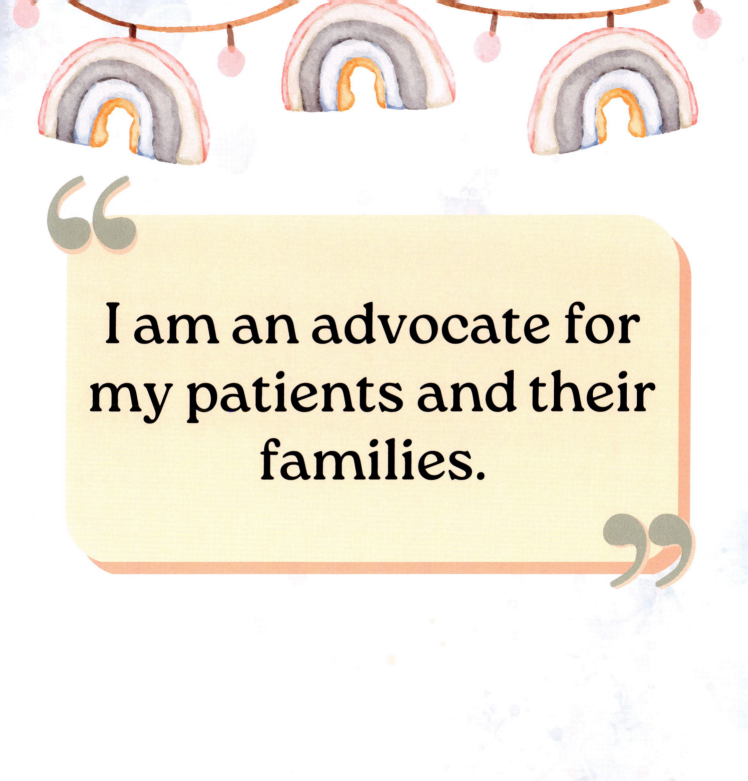

> I am an advocate for my patients and their families.

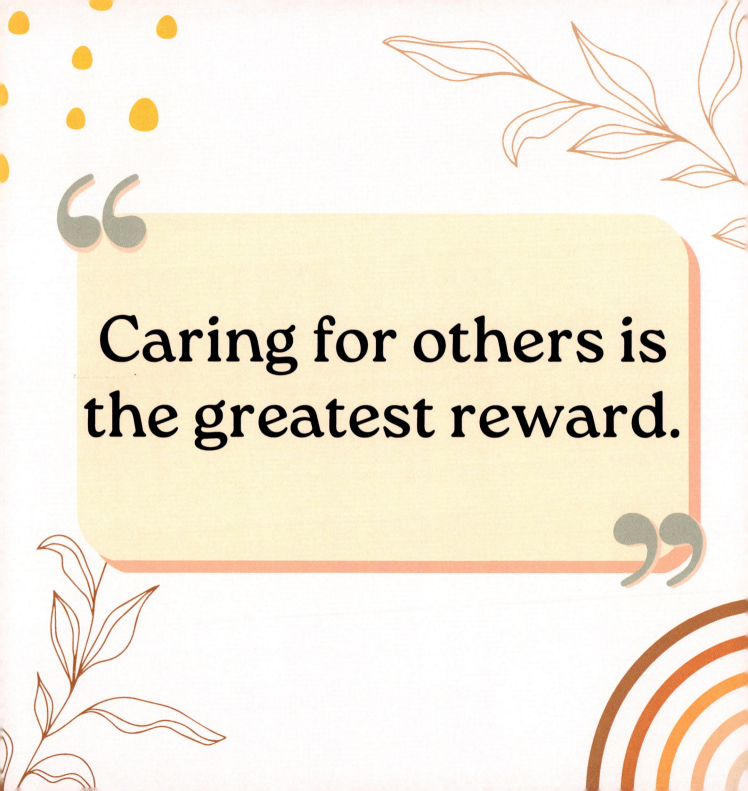

Caring for others is the greatest reward.

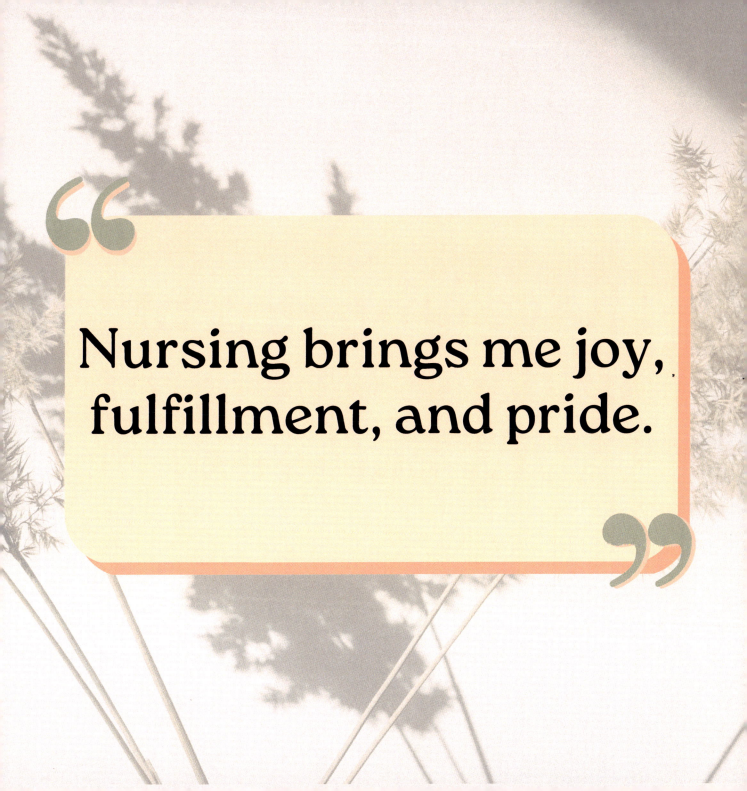

Nursing brings me joy, fulfillment, and pride.

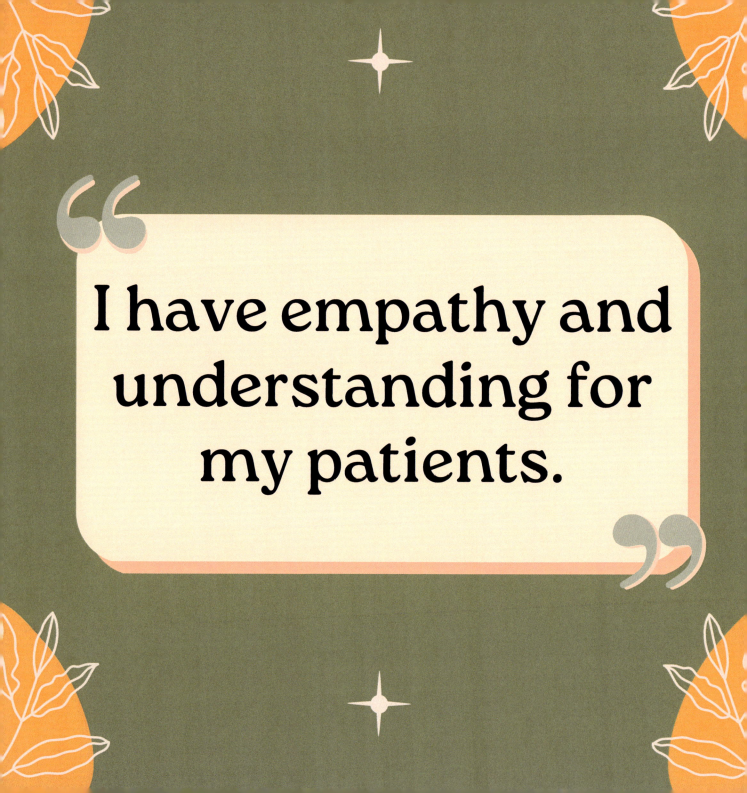

"I have empathy and understanding for my patients.

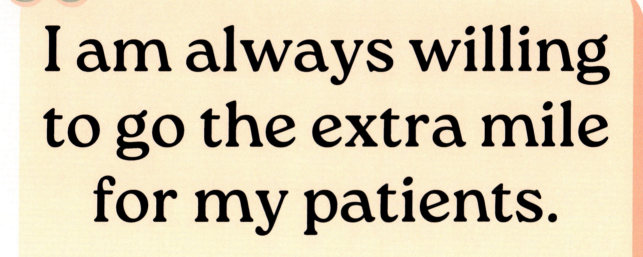

"I am always willing to go the extra mile for my patients."

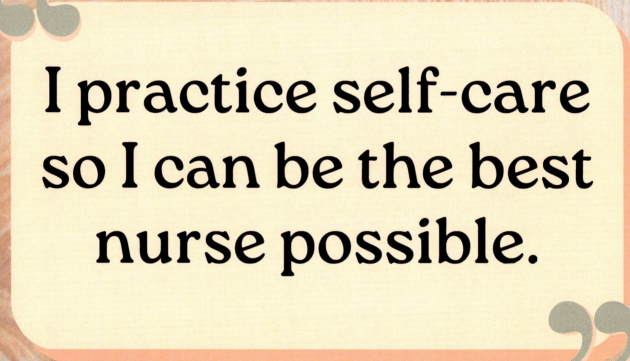

"I practice self-care so I can be the best nurse possible."

"

My work gives me purpose and meaning in life.

"

"

I am thankful that I get to do such meaningful work.

"

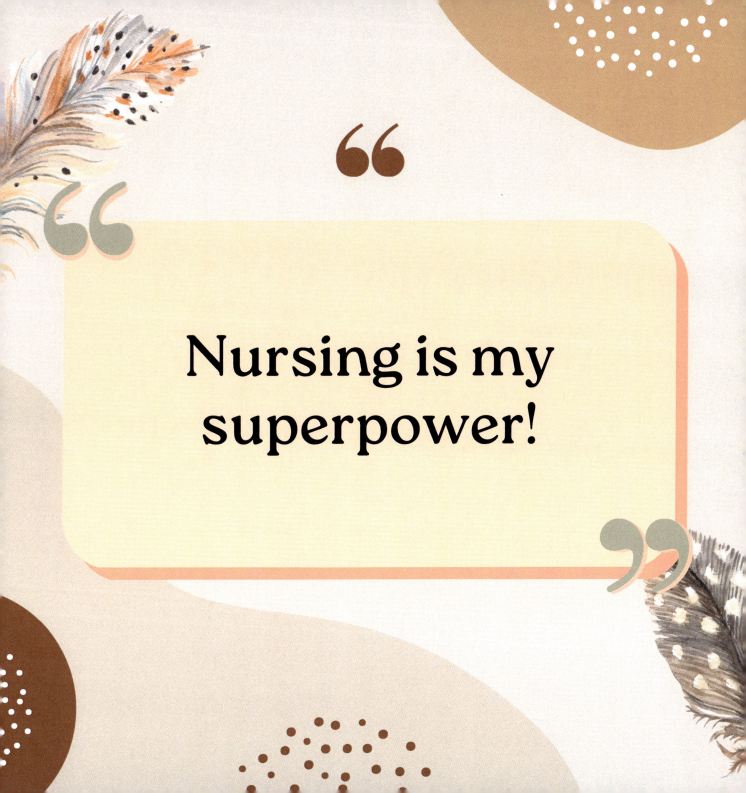

Nursing is my superpower!

I am making a difference in the world and that matters.

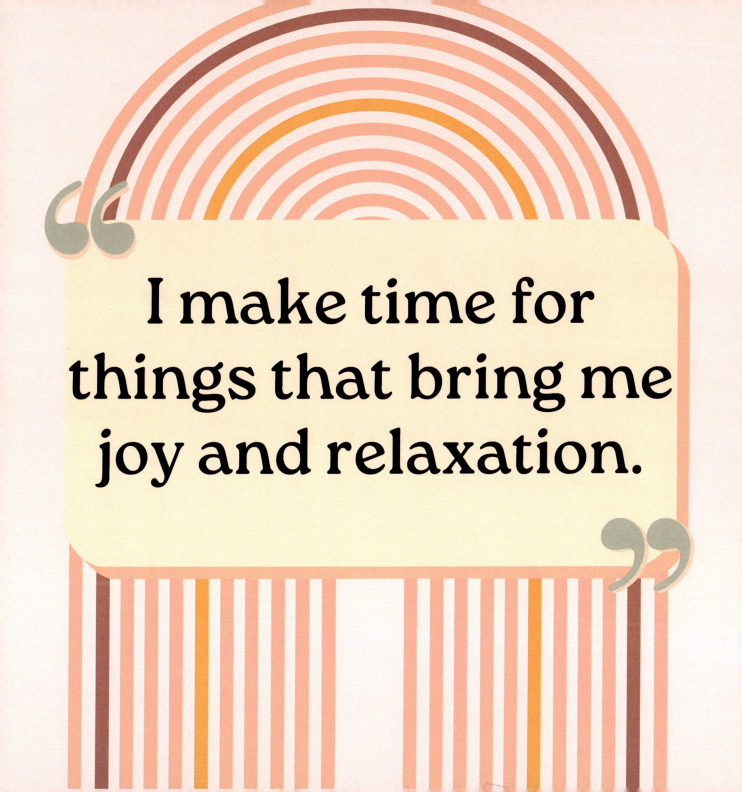

I make time for things that bring me joy and relaxation.

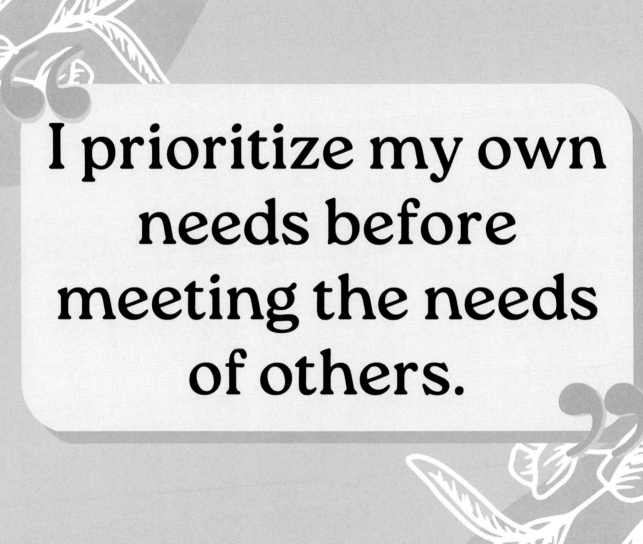

I prioritize my own needs before meeting the needs of others.

"

I seek out activities that restore and energize me.

"

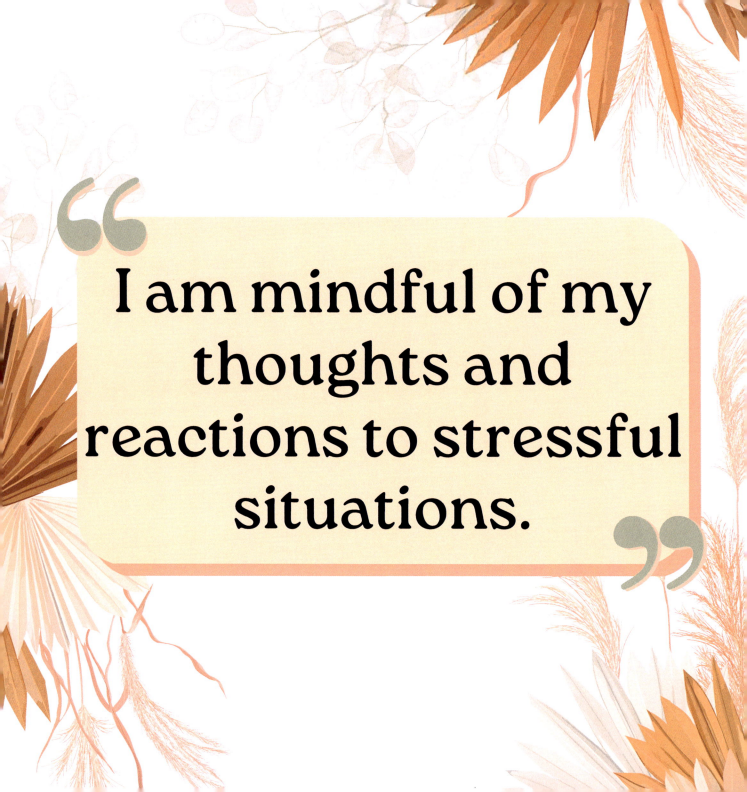

I am mindful of my thoughts and reactions to stressful situations.

I make time for meaningful conversations with friends and family.

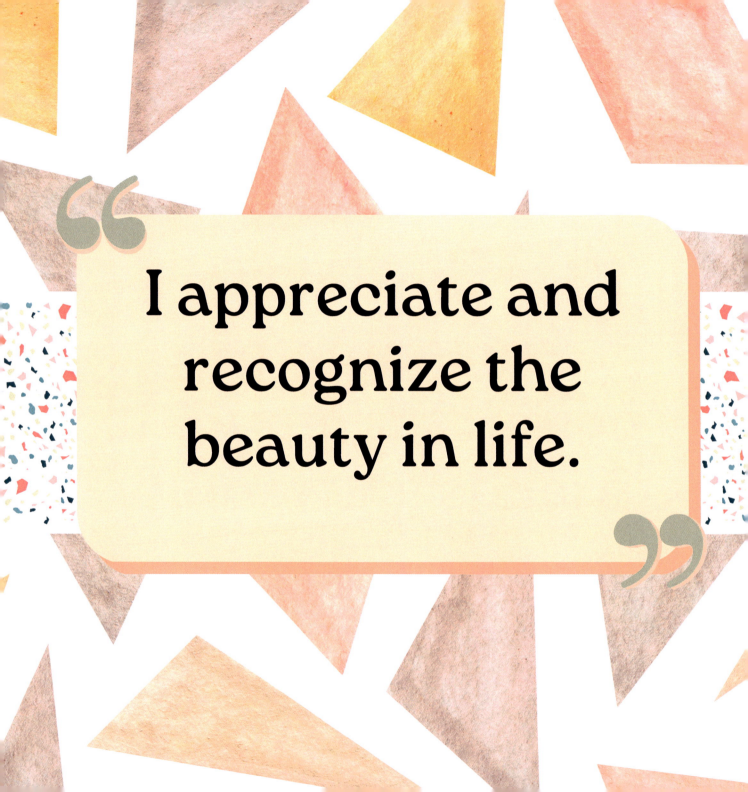

"

I appreciate and recognize the beauty in life.

"

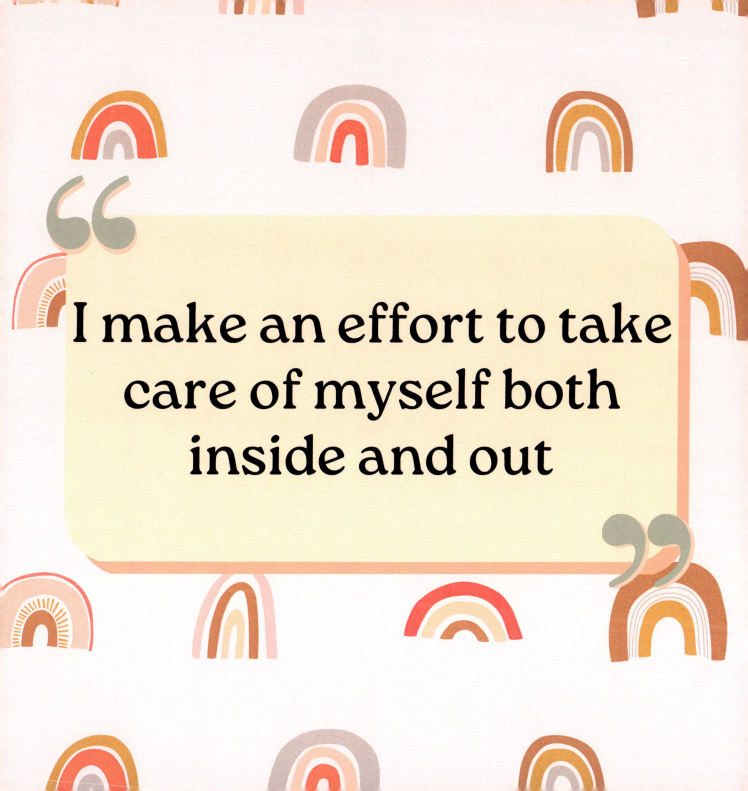

I make an effort to take care of myself both inside and out

# "

I have the confidence to handle any situation that comes my way.

**"**

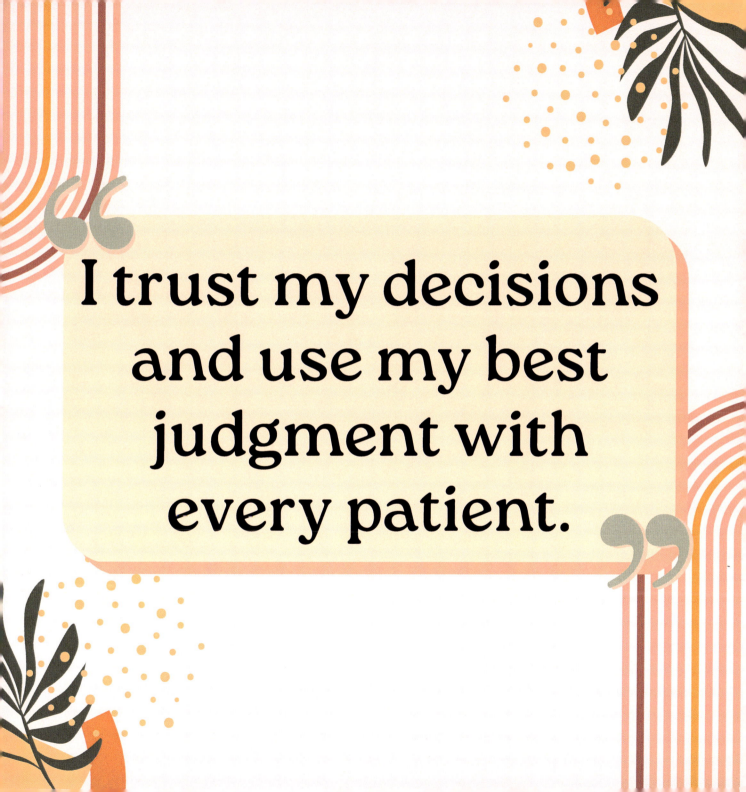

"I trust my decisions and use my best judgment with every patient."

# I believe in myself and my abilities as a nurse.

# I stay positive even in challenging situations.

Made in the USA
Monee, IL
04 May 2025